There is Another Way
Energy Medicine for Pets with Cancer

Suzanne Clegg

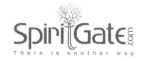

ACKNOWLEDGEMENTS

I would like to express my gratitude to William Bengston, who patiently and generously mentored me with my first cancer cures.

I am also grateful for my clients and their magnificent animal companions. It has been an honor to serve each and every one of you.

I would like to thank Fabienne Fredrickson for enthusiastically encouraging me to write this book.

Thanks to my Spirit Gate team, especially my assistant Midori Griño, for working with me on a daily basis, enabling me to publish this book.

I am grateful for my husband Ted and my daughters Abigail and Phoebe, who supported and encouraged me not only in the writing of this book, but in the many unconventional adventures with my career.

Last, but not least, I am grateful to Georgette, my hamster, as well as Nikky and Annie, my dear dogs who taught me much about how animals heal.

CONTENTS

INTRODUCTION

Does your pet have cancer? Are you aware of the benefits of energy medicine but you're not sure about how it may help cancer? Are you worried about how to care for your pet as they go through the process? You would like a cure, but comfort and manageability are also important? This book explains my method of teaching you how to activate your pet's innate healing ability. It is easy to learn and in certain situations, quite effective, even for a beginner!

You may be familiar with William Bengston, PhD's research, where in 15 peer reviewed university settings, he was able to document cancer cures in almost all of the mice that had otherwise incurable cancer. Once Bengston found he could do it, he had skeptical graduate students do his method and their mice also were cured. I cannot promise that you can cure your animal, but I can tell you I am fully trained by Bengston in his method that got these results. I have developed it into my own approach using video coaching so that your pet is relaxed. If you would like to try it, I can help you do so.

I won't be going into the fundamentals of energy medicine. I am assuming that if you are reading this, you are already familiar with some versions of it: acupuncture, laying-on-of-hands, *Reiki*, Healing Touch, prayer, etc. You already know that your pet is not just bones and blood, but also has emotions and a soul. You already know that the physical body can be affected by emotions and spiritual input and you want to include this in your care for your sick animal friend.

This method is different from most energy healing methods—I know because I have been trained in and even taught many of them. I had to unlearn much of what I "knew" about sound healing, faith healing, *Qi Gong*, shamanism, Therapeutic Touch, and acupuncture. I now integrate these methods sparingly when I am cooling down a tumor. My method overlaps with other energy medicine methods, and may at first glance seem to be working the same way, but there are important differences.

This book should give you enough information to know if this energy healing method is something you want to learn to do for your pet to boost their healing.

Be prepared to receive a deeply loving paradigm shift that will not only help your beloved animal, but you as well. All you need is your hands, an open heart, and the willingness to do the exercises.

Let's begin!

CHAPTER ONE

Six Things I Tell People When They Learn Their Pet Has Cancer

1. There is another way.

In fact, there are *lots* of other ways! This book describes my way of working with cancer using a non-invasive energy medicine method. If your pet is young (for their breed's normal lifespan) and never had chemo or radiation therapy, they are the ideal candidates for trying my method. This book will give you enough information to know if you want to use this method to help your pet.

2. You don't have to be "gifted" to help your pet.

You are off the hook! Your animal friend will get healing from the Source, not from you, so you don't have to be enlightened or extraordinarily gifted with special healing abilities. This book will *give you the confidence to touch your pet while practicing a visualization exercise in your head.* You will learn what to look for in a naturally healing tumor. You'll learn to avoid common mistakes. You will want a veterinarian on the team to share their clinical experience so your pet gets really great well-rounded care.

3. My method has a foundation of solid scientific research.

I started my cancer-healing adventures with William Bengston, PhD. Bengston did 15 different controlled University laboratory studies. He documented again and again, cancer cures in mice. He found that not only did the mice's cancer completely go away, they were also immune to the recurrence of cancer. He trained skeptical graduate students to do his method and they got similar results – their mice's cancer also was cured. He personally mentored me how to work successfully with my human cancer patients.

4. My method for pets is an extension of my work with people.

Bill Bengston generously taught me his image cycling technique and how to manage naturally-healing tumors. I learned the subtle and not-so-subtle things to pay attention to. He gave me the confidence to work with cancer. My 35 years clinical experience with Western, Chinese and Anthroposophic medicine have helped me understand how cancer-healing works and give me ideas of what to change if something is stuck. I had many teachers who taught me how to work with my clairvoyance. These all led me to be able to access my "true teacher", which is the Substance of the Universe and the True Nature of my patients.

When you learn this method, you will not need all this. All my training and experience has prepared me to help you and be your teacher. Beginners have tremendous luck with this, possibly because their Ego is out of the way. The actual technique is quite accessible to a lay person. You don't need to believe in it or even be "good" at it! All you need is an open heart, some clear thinking and the willingness to do it.

5. Be prepared for your own inner transformation as you help your pet heal.

Be prepared to receive a deeply loving paradigm shift that will not only help your beloved animal, but you as well! The first time I cured cancer, I was so happy—but it also rocked my inner world. It had been so easy! I had just followed a protocol! My patient was pretty sure he was wasting his time, and I was hopeful but rather anxious and insecure. If it was so easy to cure cancer, what about all the other things that seem impossible? I was happy my patient was better...and I was disoriented. I had been doing energy medicine as an acupuncturist, sound healer and shaman for 30 years and had never experienced anything like it! It led me to consider my life differently. It also led me to offer my experience to you in the form of this book.

I have watched similar experiences in my students who learn to help their animals. You may not have a mini "identity crisis," like I did, but I can just about promise you that some part of your psyche will be freed up. Being in the presence of a tumor healing itself almost always touches one in a profound way. It is a big deal. It's not that you necessarily have great insights into the nature of Life. You don't start levitating. It's more that when your pet gets better, it tends to lift the whole system they live in. Sometimes I wonder who is getting the more profound healing…the dog with cancer or the dog's owner.

6. Yes, this method is experimental — and you have support.

The last thing I want to do is give you false hope. There are no guarantees in life, and especially not in the cancer world. But, no guarantee *does not* mean no support. If you are learning my method, I want to know how you are doing. I did not write this book because I have healed thousands of cats and dogs. I am not the "John of God" for horses. *I am just a few steps ahead of you.* I have a researcher's mind and I want to discover what works and how to teach it. As you work with your animal you will discover things that I didn't know about the method. You will have questions for which others will have answers. If it doesn't work, I want to know about that too! I invite you to be part of a forum and support network of others trying this method. Let's take this process, practice it, and see if it can help you and your animal friend.

CHAPTER TWO

Is This You?

 I don't want to give my pet chemo!

"The vet has offered chemo as "something to do," which might make me feel less helpless, because it might extend my pet's life, but has not given me hope for a good outcome."

"The chemotherapy or radiation seems brutal. I know my pet will not live forever and I care about their quality of life."

"I can't afford the chemo or radiation but I want to do something."

"I would never treat my own cancer with poison, why would I give it to my pet?"

"My vet told me that the cancer is so advanced that the chemo is likely to not work, will be expensive, and will make my pet uncomfortable. Between the visits to the vet and nursing a sick animal, it's not a good

choice. I am not willing to sit and watch this young animal die without doing anything. I need to find another way."

Do any of those statements sound like you?

My method doesn't work magically. It doesn't defy natural laws. *It is comforting (perhaps life-extending) but not curative for an older animal or one that has had chemo or radiation.* If the animal is currently receiving chemo, it may stop the chemo from working and the chemo may stop my method from working. I don't recommend doing them at the same time.

This whole chemo issue is important, so I put some emphasis on it. It's not that I hate veterinarians or Western medicine (I don't). It's not that I am opposed to chemo or radiation for cancer (there's a time and place for everything). It's not that I haven't tried to help people and animals who have had chemo and radiation (I have).

It's because the tumors in an animal that have had the deep poisons don't respond well. A hot tumor in a young animal will dramatically cool down during a healing session. If they have had chemo, their tumor doesn't cool down (or it is a wimpy cool down, not a robust cool breeze). In Chapter 6, I'll explain how to tell if it is working. Unfortunately, older animals and animals that have had chemo or radiation therapy often don't respond much. Their tumors energetically feel like a "dead battery".

Spontaneous remissions happen frequently in cancer. They happen in people (and perhaps animals) who have had full chemo and radiation, so it is not that I don't think it is possible. This hope led me to treat many people and animals who had had chemo or radiation. I haven't had a cure this way. It has been worthwhile palliative care (they had less pain, better digestion, and seemed more cheerful), but no cures. I have some ideas of how to get around this, but it requires a group of people (healers) experienced in the Method. This book is my attempt to start training people so that such groups can form.

Is This You?

I'm comfortable with natural healing methods. But I have no clue how to help my pet with cancer.

Maybe you know *Reiki*, acupuncture, Healing Touch, laying-on-of hands faith healing, shamanism, energy psychology, ...*and* you have a much-deserved respect for the difficulty in treating cancer. You want to try what you know and learn something new, but you need guidance. If this is you, welcome.

The only risk using my method is the risk that you will rely on it and avoid something else that could have worked better. I'll teach you how to know if it is working. I will help you include your veterinarian and anyone else that will give you a helpful perspective.

Is This You?

I'm intrigued… But I have my doubts.

You know that all sorts of things are possible with energy medicine, but you may wonder if this particular method is for real. You may be skeptical about it helping you. That's ok. I'm going to go through the Method and help you work through your questions and concerns. I had all these concerns myself, so like I said before, I am just one step ahead of you. I didn't know if I could do it. I didn't know if I had the time. I thought that Bengston had a magical touch. I didn't know how to really tell if I was being effective or not. I didn't know how frequently to treat. I didn't know where to touch or how hard to press. I didn't know how to get my Ego out of the way and do "nothing" while I was doing "something." I didn't know what to do if the animal wasn't interested. I didn't know how to explain to my family why it was suddenly so important for me to do this. If you have your doubts, and are willing to keep an open mind, welcome!

Is This You?

I don't believe you! This is ridiculous!

You may be feeling vulnerable and sense that you are being given false hope. You may not even know what "energy medicine" is! You are just looking into this because you don't want your young pet to die—she's your best friend and you'd do anything for her! You are stressed out with your pet's condition and have your doubts about taking on a whole different way of looking at the cancer.

You worry that I may be a very well-meaning, but deluded person. You don't trust science, so Bengston's research results don't motivate you to investigate.

If this is you, please do not waste your time. This approach is not for everyone. This book will not teach you the fundamentals of energy medicine—you will have to go elsewhere for that. This book is mostly for people who are already looking for something like this, who are familiar with healing without drugs or surgery and want some guidance. There are many other ways to help your pet. Follow your heart and your gut and your clear thinking to find what fits you.

My students usually feel a deep sense of connection, of destiny, of being guided by "coincidences" to this work. When they work with me, they feel like they are coming home to a part of themselves that they have always wanted to develop. It feels "important" to them to work this way with their pet.

My students know that they are working against the odds. They feel drawn to this work, it makes sense, and they I want to give it a try. If you have a relatively young animal with cancer who has never had chemo or radiation therapy, I think you should give it a try. I will teach you things to notice that reassure you if you are on the right track and help you know if nothing is happening.

This book is a summary of the major points in the Method. To really do the technique, most people need some sort of coaching. I can coach you online privately or with a group. I love computer video coaching. I can see you and your pet, but your pet is not disturbed by my physical presence. I don't treat animals (I am not a vet). I only educate pet owners how to treat their pets themselves.

Please do not confuse my enthusiasm for hype. It's poignantly real to me that this method is experimental. I've treated people and animals that died in spite of my best efforts. I learned from each of them. I want to spare you some of my learning curve. I don't regret working with them. I think it was an important chapter in both of our lives. That being said, I offer you a systematic method of energy healing that you can use on your pet, and likely succeed even as a beginner.

CHAPTER THREE

My Vision

A foundational part of this method is the use of powerful positive images. The method is not *just* positive imaging, but it is a crucial piece. When you become my student, I want you to succeed. I want us to succeed. I have a picture in my mind of what I hope for. It may or may not happen, but I am clear that I want it. My Vision may change as I get to know you and as I train more students, but for now, this is what I imagine:

My Vision for You

It is six months from now and your pet is cancer free. They are healthy and strong. There is a twinkle in their eyes, a lilt in their gait. They are not weakened, but rather strengthened from their bout with cancer. You and your family aren't worried about your pet's health. You are spending your time doing all sorts of things unrelated to their condition, because there is no condition. You have a document framed on the wall. It is letter from your veterinarian certifying that your pet had cancer and is now cancer free. Perhaps someone who knows how your pet was cured needs help with their pet. You can offer it…or not, but your "cancer terror" is now "cancer concern" and you are free to act out of love. You've changed, too. You feel more like "yourself" than you used to. It's as if the whole cancer episode allowed something inside you to "finish" or "complete". You feel a little more Present to your life. You now embody a certain wisdom and ability to trust in the process of life that is deeper than before.

My Vision for Us

It's a year from now. While you were learning to help your animal, we got to know each other. Maybe you joined my group video coaching and you also know others who were also learning to help their animals. You sent me a letter from your vet certifying the cancer remission. Your pet's photo is on the "Healing Tree". This is an artist's drawing of a tree with lots of circles all over it. The circles have different colors: gold, silver, copper, etc. Inside the circles with the gold frames are the photos of the people with their pets that have been cured. Not everyone who is attracted to this method is going to have a young chemo-free animal -- I want your story and photo too! If you feel the method helped your beloved pet with their condition, let's celebrate that success as well! Once we have hundreds of photos on this tree, I envision the "100th Monkey" effect happening, and suddenly the whole paradigm around cancer care collapses, implodes on itself (similar to how a tumor acts when it heals). Fast forward a few decades. A youngster looks incredulously at you when you tell them how cancer used to be treated. You smile and know that you and your beloved animal companion were part of that transformation. It feels good.

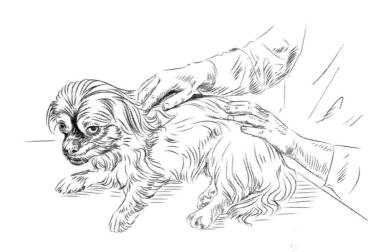

Annie being treated

CHAPTER FOUR

What Is This Method?

It is an observation-based method — not a faith-based method. You touch your pet with your hands while activating certain thoughts and being very aware of subtle emotional and physical shifts. It is an energy medicine approach that honors the resonance between the physical, life force, emotions, imagination and spiritual aspects of the animal and their "person".

On the Physical Level

You are comfortably touching your animal friend with your hands. I take the idea of "laying-on-of-hands" very literally— your hands are gently touching your pet. Your cat or small dog can be on your lap. If you have a hamster or bird that is in a cage, you can simply hold the cage with your hands. You can do the technique while you are grooming your horse.

On the Life Force Level

You are noticing the *Qi* or the sense of vitality, warmth, coolness, activity or non-activity in your pet. You will also want to notice your own life force. Make sure that your *Hara* (deep inside lower abdomen just below navel) and your heart are just as present with the process as your head and your hands are. You want to be contained in your own body and your own life force. You are in no way trying to transfer life force from your body to your pet.

On the Emotional Level

You are noticing your own feelings, your pet's feelings. You will want to connect lovingly with your pet — not the sentimental oozy energy-sucking love, rather a grounded open heart willing to be helpful in their healing process. During the treatment, you and your pet may have a variety of emotions arise. These are important and should be experienced with interest.

On the Imagination Level

You will be focusing on two things at once. The first is doing the *Clegg Resonance Cycling Technique*, which I teach in my classes. If you'd like to learn more about this and get a free copy of the basics, just send me an email at *info@spiritgate.com* and let me know.

The second is that you want to imagine that you can see inside your pet's body. Most people will not succeed at actually being able to see what is in there, but the very act of pretending that you can see is therapeutic. The inner gesture of connecting to the inside of your pet with your imagination creates a special connection that I find helps beginners succeed at cooling down their pets' tumors.

Your imagination and emotions link you to the spiritual dimensions that contain the information your pet needs to heal. I have been working energetically with people for so many years that my ability to perceive emotions stored in the body comes to me in the form of images. I am able to "tune in" to your pet and notice if they are "receiving" the information they need for healing. I can do this in person, over the phone or Skype. I teach my students how to adjust their hand position so that their pet receives the healing. This skill helps me teach and treat, but my students do not need to do this. It's about their animal's process, and there are plenty of non-intuitive clues that will let you know if you are on the right track.

On the Spiritual Level

The actual healing comes from supra-conscious "place" that you are unconscious of. Thoughts and images may *come from* this place, but they are not the source of the information. I call that supra-conscious, non-physical place "Source".

I like to consider that my pet has a spiritual dimension. I think of the individuality of my pet as well as their species. For example, if I am healing my dog Annie, I am aware of my love and delight in her, I am aware of her beautiful fur and her loving eyes, I am aware of her unique individuality. Then I go *through* all that and touch with my consciousness, her "dogness". If I was working on a cat, I would connect with her *through* her individuality to the way she is the same as any other cat. I do not do this when I work on people as we are naturally more separate from each other than animals are with their species.

Not all thinking is the same. Ego-centered thinking, which most of our thinking is, does *not* create the healing — it gets in the way. Usually any thought that assumes you are doing the healing, that the healing is coming "through" you, that you have to "inwardly align with a positive outcome" will get in the way. My *Clegg Resonance Cycling Technique* is a wonderful decoy for your ego. If you are a beginner, it really is quite effective at getting your ego out of the way. I developed this technique using my own spiritual research of William Bengston's image cycling technique. You can learn from both approaches. The differences are in how I teach it, how fast people are able to begin healing effectively, ways I play with it, and the various philosophic containers I put the technique in.

Soon, with a little practice, you become comfortable with the *Clegg Resonance Cycling Technique* and will be able to do it while you talk, walk and think of other things. At that point, it will be a less effective decoy for your ego. You will continue to do the technique but need something else to do with your mind. You will want to use your mind in the "receiving and observing" mode—not the "making something happen" mode. While you do the cycling technique in the back of your mind, you will use the front of your mind to *simply and carefully observe* how your pet is responding to the information that she is receiving from Source. You will use your thinking to notice if it is time to change your hand position, to cycle at a different speed, to do nothing, or something else. When you are observing something without directing it, you are present but detached. That's what you want.

This may seem confusing but it becomes simple and do-able with online video coaching. Promise!

During the video coaching you will be physically touching your pet. I will be touching your pet with my Intention while doing a Distance Healing and talking to you. I can cool down tumors remotely, but it works much better if there are some human hands on the animal. Physical comfort and physical changes are closely observed as they help us adjust the non-physical things we do. The Method is not just about enhancing the Life Force. It's not about getting a sense of "flow", nor a "magnetic feeling". It's not even about the cooling down of a tumor. These things happen as a *result* of the healing, but are not the healing.

If you want to increase the power of the healing, it is tempting to combine it with acupuncture, sound healing, and other healing methods. If nothing is happening, I may use other energy methods to "get things started", but then less really is more!

My method is so subtle that as soon as I start directing the energy in any way, I actually interfere with the innate wisdom. I have observed this in cancer more than in other conditions. The best way I have found to amplify a healing is to work as a team with two or more people treating the animal at once.. For example, if your hands are on your pet and I am connecting remotely on the phone or Skype, it helps boost things a lot. Together, we are usually better than either one of us alone.

Emotional healing is always part of any physical healing. It can be quite dramatic with cancer. Animals have their own emotional issues and they can take on and hold in their bodies, the toxic emotions of the people they care about. My method addresses or clears emotional interference differently than psychotherapy and spiritual counseling (which don't really apply to animals). In my coaching I help people know how it feels to have an emotion "leaving the tissue" that it was attached to. I help you do the *Clegg Resonance Cycling Technique* when you experience strong emotion. One of the reasons I think it is so much easier to treat animals than people is that they are attached to their emotions very differently than we are, and it's easier for them to let go of emotional negativity.

Many types of energy medicine, prayer, and laying-on-of-hands include religion. They create a very beautiful spiritual container for their work. My method is different. I respect religion and I love philosophy, but they are mental containers for consciousness.

The place that healing comes from cannot be contained in a box. I'm not saying we shouldn't have religions. I'm not saying that we shouldn't devise systems to explain the non-physical. I'm saying that the healing comes from a dimension that is beyond all that. You don't align yourself with the correct religious/philosophic perspective to get a cure... It happens the other way around. As a result of curing your cat from cancer, your religious/philosophic box will get bigger and truer. You will have a perspective that you didn't have before. You cannot shift something in you to force Grace, but when Grace is received, everything shifts.

This method is about honoring the wholeness of something, so it really can be used to treat anything. While I was writing this chapter, I took a break and used the method on a tree in my yard. The tree had a huge branch pruned from it earlier in the day. I sensed it could use some healing. I don't think the tree has cancer, but I did feel an energetic shift similar to a tumor cooling down. I sensed information entering the tree that will be helpful. It felt like a "block" of information emerging — as if it was already there but the tree wasn't connecting to it. I got a subtle sense of relief and happiness as something re-integrated.

This book is about helping animals with cancer because it is easy for me to coach people remotely, over the phone or Skype, how to manage a naturally healing tumor. I'm not so sure what to expect from the tree, or from a business that needs healing.

What about treating an animal with a non-cancerous health problem? I would say go for it, give it a try, but each condition will have its own way of healing, so you may need more medical knowledge than most people have. It's paradoxical that cancer, which physical medicine finds so hard to treat, is so easy to teach a lay person how to help. I have a lot of ideas about why cancer may be easier than back pain, which I take up in my coaching programs.

My group coaching will be restricted to mammals that can have a camera aimed at them during the class so everyone else can see what is happening. That means mostly dogs, cats, and rodents in cages. I have some experience working with horses, and I am itching to help a horse person help their friend. I'm sure birds and snakes would respond, but I have not worked with many, and don't know what to tell you to look for in how their tumors heal, so we would have to explore that individually.

When I say that the method "works," I don't mean that it will always "cure". If your pet is old, has had chemo or doesn't have a rapidly growing tumor, you might not get a dramatic response. In Chapter 6, you will learn how to tell if you are on the right track.

Can you do this?
What preparation do you need?

If you are attracted to this work, you can probably do it. It helps to be sensitive, but that's just a perk. All you really need is interest and the willingness to practice. The only preparation is to get an overview, which you are doing by reading this book, and start. Just like learning anything else, be prepared for some beginners luck, a stuck place that you have to work through, and then a release into confidence. If you need help, don't hesitate to contact me at *info@spiritgate.com*.

CHAPTER FIVE

Healing with Your Heart, Hara, Hands & Head

At last! We have arrived at what to actually DO and THINK and FEEL during a healing session.

Step One. Opening with the Heart and the Hara

Before you even approach your pet, center yourself in your heart. Most of us walk around and are not embodied. If you ask us where we are, we say "in the thing I was just reading", or "all over the place", or "in the past", or "in the future." To begin a healing session, it helps if you are in your body and in the here and now. Do a body check. Feel the weight of your body connecting with your chair or the ground. Notice any tightness or relaxation in your body. Notice any anxiety or peace. Notice... Notice... Notice. Notice if you tend to skip this step, and gently return to it if you did.

Create a boundary or a spiritual container for the exercise. Simply say to yourself, "I am now going to practice this healing procedure with [*name of your pet*]." Some people pray and ask that the room be a safe place for receiving healing. One of my favorite prayers is, "I open my heart to the possibility of healing." You might imagine a circle of healing light around you and your pet. You can do whatever invocation you want. Some sort of personally authentic opening is helpful, so experiment with what feels best to you.

Now acknowledge your physical body, especially the middle of your chest, (your heart area) and your *Hara* (your lower abdomen). Don't try to manufacture any particular sensation, just bring your attention to heart and your *Hara*. Be aware of your whole body, and invite extra awareness to your heart and *Hara*.

Feel the beating of your heart and the quiet of your *Hara*.

It helps to hold still and do this, but with animals that is not always an option. You can be aware of your body even if you are in motion. You are going to try to keep the awareness of your Heart and *Hara* during the whole session. This helps you stay contained in yourself, and allows your pet the freedom to heal in their own way and in their own time.

Step Two: Scan for Emotions

Scanning for emotions is like walking outside and noticing if it is hot, cold, windy or humid. What is the emotional "weather" in the room? In you? In your animal friend? This is a base-line reading that you notice, so that if something

24

changes you will be able to observe it. Don't judge the emotions. It's always OK to make yourself or your animal more comfortable—physically or emotionally. If your dog is just sitting there, minding his own business, you might not get a strong emotional reading on him. If you are aware of your own emotions and the emotional weather in the room, as the session progresses, and if an emotional issue that is in your dog's tissue is released, you may feel it in yourself or in the room. When cancer heals naturally, the emotional history sometimes goes backwards and you get a whiff of what emotions went into the cancer as they leave.

If you have trouble, just pretend that you can tell what you and your pet are feeling. You can tell when you walk into a room if there has been a recent argument—it's the same thing with sensing the emotions in your pet. If you pay attention, and with some practice, you can also feel happiness, sadness, and anger. There is not always a lot of emotion at the beginning of a treatment, so don't worry if you don't feel much. You are not so interested in what is there, as much as what *changes* during the session.

You can sense emotional shifts in a variety of ways. Stay relaxed and centered in your vertical axis, your heart and *Hara* throughout the session as you observe any changes in the emotional weather of the room, of you or your pet.

Step Three: Make Energetic Contact

Arrange yourself and your pet so you can touch them. Place a few of your right hand fingers lightly on your pet anywhere that it is easy to reach. Use your left hand with slightly relaxed fingers, to pass over your animal's energy field. This is usually a few inches off their body although for horses it can be several feet. Notice if there are areas of a magnetic pull or push, areas of hot or cold, areas that seem to want you to touch them, and areas that seem to not want to be touched. Don't worry if you are right or wrong, it doesn't work that way. Don't worry if you are making it up. If you are a beginner to feeling the energy field around your pet's body, it works just fine to fake it until you make it. If I were to watch you doing this over Skype, we would both sense at the same time something "important" about a certain spot on your pet. Watching others in the group video call work with their animals will give you confidence that what you are feeling is real.

If your pet is in a cage (as in a hamster), place the cage on your lap or on a table that you are sitting at. You can scan the cage with your hand to determine hot/cold, push/pull, want/don't want, almost as if the cage was the "body" of your pet. Watch my YouTube video *Hamster Healed with Energy Medicine* to see how I placed my hands on Georgette's cage.

At this stage of sensing with your hand, since you are not really touching the physical body yet, do include your heart and other parts of your body in your sensing. You are not trying to do anything but notice what is. Since your heart is open, this sensing can be a loving connection, but avoid sentimentality. Gushy gooey love is usually more about you and not about a genuine connection with another.

Horses have enormous energy fields... Usually 12 feet away from the body! You will probably sense with your whole body where the edge is. You don't have to be "at the edge", or anywhere in particular... Just be where it feels right today.

Four-legged mammals are, as a rule, more grounded than upright people. Sense their grounding. Stay in your *Hara* so you can observe from a grounded place inside yourself.

Step 4. Making Physical Contact

Once you are exquisitely tuned in to where your pet's energy field welcomes your touch, place your hands there. Then check the tumor area. Notice if there is heat coming from the tumor. This is important, as it is best to treat when the tumor is hot. You want to become very familiar with the heat of your animal's tumor. It's easy to tell with a superficial tumor. It's harder with a deep one. Leukemia travels about, but there are hot spots that may appear in different locations on different days. If the tumor is deep inside the body where you can't feel its heat, I can help you find other ways to determine if it is a good time to treat. You can't over-treat, so just treat frequently if you can't tell.

Once you have inspected the energy field and the physical sense of temperature, return to that place that felt so right to touch. If you are new to feeling for energy fields, just put your left hand on their lower back. Use your left hand (which is controlled mostly by your intuitive right brain) as the treating hand. Then touch anywhere convenient with your right hand, or a finger-or-two of your right hand. My right hand is a "ground". There are no rules, but in general I like to initially place my left hand in a spot that is *not* the tumor area. In my coaching program I can help you find the right spots if you are insecure. It's a lot easier with video contact! There is no "wrong" place to touch your pet. There are just "good" and "better" places. Don't fret about being in the wrong spot, but do try to notice if one spot feels better than another and try to spend some time there.

Step 5. Start your Clegg Resonance Cycling Technique

This you can read about ahead of time and you then use the time while you are touching your pet to practice it. This technique has you mentally attach and then detach from physical things, life force phenomenon, emotions, images and then even thoughts. It's a whole process that takes practice but you need to start somewhere. You don't have to be good at it for it to be therapeutically effective. It is my experience that progress in learning the technique is more important than how good you are at it—at least at first.

If you are a beginner, simply pretend that you have a propeller attached to a cap on your head and it is spinning so fast that the propeller is a blur. Keep this spinning, moving image in your head while you touch your pet. You may forget that you are supposed to be thinking this thought, so like any meditation, bring yourself back to it. Return and return.

Notice that you can be aware of what your hands are feeling *while* you are spinning the imaginary propeller on your head. Notice how you can be aware of emotional shifts *while* you are spinning your propeller.

I intend to write a whole book just about the *Clegg Resonance Cycling Technique*, but I am deliberately not going into a larger explanation now so that as a beginner, you keep it simple. You can start cooling down your pet's tumor just by imagining a propeller spinning on your head while touching them. There is more to it than this, and it may not be enough for a thorough cure, but it gets you started and gets your confidence up. If you are ready for the specifics of how to take the mental technique past a simple spinning propeller, simply email *info@spiritgate.com* and I'll send you detailed written or audio instructions and how to get coaching on it.

Step 6. Move your hands to a different spot

After a minute or so, you will get the sense that it is time to move your hands to a new spot. Repeat the process of feeling the energy field with your left hand until it gets to a spot it likes. Place your *right* hand in a spot that makes your *left* hand feel more "active". You continue holding and then moving until the tumor has cooled down and you feel a cool breeze over the tumor area. If you have a young animal with a rapidly growing tumor, this cooling is NOT subtle. You don't need your intuition—your hand feels a chill instead of warmth coming from the tumor area. It rarely happens in a flash. It usually takes 5-30 minutes for a tumor to cool down. The more rapidly growing the tumor is, the more it responds with this cool down. Slow growing tumors, dormant tumors, or fast-growing tumors in animals that once had chemo or radiation, don't respond enthusiastically.

Step 7. Heal the whole animal

Now that I've told you about that nifty trick, I don't want you to fixate on it. There is more to curing cancer than cooling down a tumor. It is one convenient indicator that your pet is "taking the treatment" or "receiving the spiritual information it needs to be whole again." You may feel sensations of flow while you are touching… Go with them and find places to put your hands where there seems to be more flow. You can willfully create a flow, as any *Qi Gong* practitioner can tell you. *Do not do that with this technique*, as it will interfere. You may get magnetic feelings in your hands and they may heat up. Your sensations are quite irrelevant to your pet's healing process. Sorry. I wish I could say that hotter hands mean more healing, but that's not the way it works. Simply notice what you notice and keep the attention on what your pet seems to need. It's about their process not yours. Your ability to perceive and even unconsciously respond to your pet's healing process may keep you interested but should not be confused with the power that heals.

Your inner attitude is one of offering, not of fixing. Your presence helps your pet connect with something in its true nature that it is otherwise cut off from. Your touch allows your pet to receive healing direct from the Source (not through you and not from you).

Step 8. Don't give the cancer a lot of attention

You don't want to psychically attack the cancer cells. This is a big-time inappropriate use of your ego and it can feed the cancer. The cancerous cells are also your beloved pet's cells and when they remember their truth, they will die on their own. If you find yourself enraged with the cancer, don't suppress your anger but feel it *while* doing the *Clegg Resonance Cycling Technique*. In my coaching I spend time modeling inner gestures that help you be Present with the cancer without getting caught up with it. The *Clegg Resonance Cycling Technique* acts as a buffer so that the healing happens even if you don't have the perfect inner attitude.

You may have feelings of fear, revulsion, deep sadness and anger if you care about your pet. When you touch their tumor, it's common for these feeling to rise. Don't suppress them, but make sure you are spinning your imaginary propeller while you are feeling them.

Sometimes I get a strong emotion of loving gratitude and reverence while I treat. This is not usually directed at the consciousness of the cancer, rather the consciousness of the intact part of the animal that cancer can never negate. I don't "love" the tumor, but I do lovingly invite the cancer cells to remember how to receive the healing that is the primordial foundation of their true nature.

Step 9. Ending the session

If you are a beginner and can't feel energy and your animal's tumor is deep or if your animal is in a cage and you are not checking its temperature, it may be hard to know how long to treat. Let's narrow it down to a few things to think about. Soon you will be getting some sort of "click" when it's time to stop.

- Some treatment is better than no treatment. A 30-second treatment is better than no treatment.

- It's hard to treat too much. It doesn't seem to hurt to keep treating even if your pet has already got what it needs for now. I healed my hamster by treating her for about 5 minutes a day, and sometimes skipping days. Bengston's skeptical graduate students healed their mice by doing his rapid imaging technique while holding the mice's cage for 30 minutes a day.

- Short frequent sessions may be better than a long extended session, so keep that as a possibility. I like to think of a hot tumor as being "hungry" for healing. When it's not hot, or after it has cooled down, it is not hungry, so it doesn't do much to keep feeding it healing. Wait until it gets hungry for more.

- Cancer is chaotic by nature, so it is sure to need different amounts of time on different days.

- Start with 15 minutes and go up or down in time as you become more familiar with your pet's response.

- Often your pet will just move away when the treatment is done. This can be tricky because you need to distinguish between your pet moving away because you are annoying him with your aggressive healing style (in which case your ego is too involved and I can help you get it out of the way) or your pet is loving, loving, loving the treatment and then moves away because she is "done". This last one is good.

- The gold standard of how long a treatment lasts is to "treat until it is done". There is a characteristic settled quality, a lack of "hunger" from the energy field when it is done. If you know what to look for, it is not usually subtle and even beginners can tell.

Step 10. What to notice between sessions

Notice changes in sleep, eating, elimination, mood or mobility. In my classes, I teach you to energetically charge cotton and some simple distance healing techniques to support your pet between sessions. You may also purchase charged cotton from me if you prefer.

CHAPTER SIX

How To Tell If It's Working

This technique may seem to rely on "magical thinking," but you won't be able to tell if it is working and won't be able to make the teeny tiny adjustments in your form if you are busy thinking that it is magical. A hundred years ago, most people thought that airplanes flying people around was impossible. Now, we have schools teaching mechanics and engineers the basics. Newer and better flying machines are being developed all the time.

The same goes with my technique. The results may seem to defy the laws of nature, but since the technique is reproducible and teachable, there might be some laws we are overlooking! I don't understand all the ins and outs of how it works, but I do know what to look for. I'm OK with that. My father was an electrical engineer who didn't know what electricity was, but he invented a light that hasn't burnt out in over 30 years. Most researchers know that they are "exploring" and the mystery of it all is awe-inspiring and fun. I invite you to take on a "research" mentality.

When your pet's body heals from cancer, there will be signs that it is happening on physical, life force, emotional and spiritual levels. Below is a handy checklist that covers the common signals that healing is happening.

On the Physical Level

- Tumor cools during treatment. You may feel a cool breeze over the tumor area.
- Blood tests and scans ordered by veterinarian will indicate progress.
- Fever. Do not give medication to reduce fever. Almost every healing tumor has a stage where there is fever.
- Tumor gets larger and softer. This one can be scary—a good reason to get support from me. Veterinarians often have experience with a naturally healing tumor and can share their clinical experience.
- Tumor shrinks and disappears (sometimes within days)
- Tumor extrudes itself from the body and falls off, or can be easily cut off by a vet.

On the Life Force Level

When you are treating your pet, the energy field around the pet will "respond". Typical ways include:

- A clear sensation of "connection" and "magnetic flow".

- Your pet likes being treated. They often move away when they are done.

- Your pet starts being more active if they were lethargic. There is a lightness and lilt to their gait that was missing before.

- They become more settled if they were hyperactive.

- They sleep better, eat better and poop better.

- Their fur looks better. They are having more "good hair days."

- The light in their eyes seems brighter.

It is quite easy to create a connection and to create a magnetic-flow sensation while you are touching you pet. Be careful. This is a sign you are energetically connected, but not necessarily a sign of healing. This flow is ideally a response to something that is beyond your conscious control. If you "created" it, there may well be a healthy effect for your pet, but it won't cure cancer. "Sending" love through you to your pet may help them, comfort them and reduce their pain, but it doesn't cure cancer. Love is important but you also need to be detached. Don't use love as a tool. Just open your heart to the possibility of healing while distracting your ego with the *Clegg Resonance Image Cycling Technique*. Wait and witness the flow... Find the flow... Get happy when the flow arrives. Do not force a flow and do not mistake the flow for healing, as it depends on the source of the flow. You don't want the source to be your ego. We have to learn how to get our ego out of the way. Keeping a piece of your awareness in your

Hara (lower abdomen) also keeps you safe and keeps you from interfering. I don't think you can "pick up" cancer from your pet, but you might be more ungrounded and disorganized than you need to be afterwards. Being grounded is good for you and good for the treatment.

You know your pet has finished "taking" the treatment when they feel energetically calm, their tumor is cool and energetically quiet, and not much "flow" is happening between your hands. After the treatment wash your hands in running water. Release any energy you no longer need right down the drain. Occasionally my left hand (my active treating hand) feels "wonky" after the treatment. Rinsing in cool water returns it to its normal state. It's good to do this wash even if you don't think you need to.

On the Level of Emotions

You can expect a sudden shift, positive or negative, in your emotional state or in your animal's. Every treatment is unique so the only rule is that if there is a sudden shift in emotion, it may be coming from the healing that is happening.

- Peace Packages. I get a download, as if a chunk of information arrived, and it feels like a wave of Peace just entered the room. Trying to manufacture a peaceful feeling to induce healing usually backfires as the ego is involved. Often the tumor cools down – at least partly after a wave of positive emotion enters.

- You get happy. One of my favorite things to do is to sit with a big hot ugly tumor, because I can almost guarantee that I will get to piggyback on the happiness my patient feels when it heals.

- Negative emotion. If you are particularly grumpy after a treatment, you may be getting a whiff of the emotions that left your pet's body and are still around in the energetic field. Cancer can be caused by emotional information stored in the body. Your animal may have taken it on from people or experienced from their own trauma. It is a good sign that the treatment is working if you feel it as it leaves. Not everyone feels this but if you do, it's not a bad sign. Use Intention to clear it out of you and the room (astral debris responds to astral cleaning).

- If you experience strong positive or negative emotion during or right after the treatment be Present with it. This means you are aware with loving concern from your heart, the quietness of your *Hara,* and the spinning of your imaginary propeller while doing something with your hands.

- Some of your most tender, pure loving thoughts can unfortunately be vehicles for your Ego to interfere with the healing. For example, reverence is nice but is not a goal. Reverence is an emotion that often accompanies genuine spiritual experiences. I would describe my healing method as being "spiritual" in that it comes from a place beyond emotions and images. *Any* emotion may accompany a genuine spiritual experience, so the indicator that a spiritual experienced just happened is *not* the presence of any particular emotion. I am reverent when something happens that evokes a feeling of reverence. Reverence often emerges in me when I appreciate beauty, or when a package of peace unloads into my patient, or when a tumor cools down. I don't get reverent so I can boss God around and make things happen that I want. It doesn't work that way. Reverence doesn't create beauty...beauty creates reverence. Reverence doesn't create a healing tumor, but a healing tumor can certainly create reverence in me! A healing tumor can also create laughter or tears or something else.

- It is good mental hygiene to think thoughts that create positive emotions in us. When doing a formal healing session, however, I like to use my emotional sensitivity to sense what is happening rather than manufacture a certain emotional response. So for the duration of the treatment, I simply notice my emotions and when they get strong, I turn on my *Clegg Resonance Cycling Technique*. Tumors have cooled down when I experience transcendent light and love, as well as when I experience sadness, rage and fear.

On the Spiritual Level

You feel Nothing. This is different from the non-dualistic altered state of awareness of enlightenment. That level of expertise is not required. You just feel like yourself.

The emotional, life force and physical feedback is there, but you are connected and you are just you. You are sitting there, connected enough with your pet to appreciate that they are "taking" the healing, but you are not doing anything. You feel "nothing" in the sense that you are not trying to manipulate your pet's experience. You are just there, touching them or their cage. At first, you need to concentrate on your cycling, your loving heart, your quiet *Hara* while touching something meaningful with your hands. After a while, doing all these simultaneously becomes semi-automatic. You can be watching TV or talking politics while you are present in this manner. As long as it doesn't stop your pet from taking the healing, it's good.

You do feel "something" in the sense that you can tell healing is happening, but you are clearly not doing it... Your pet is doing the healing. Many beginners are not aware of this level of feedback. They might not be able to tell that healing is happening as it is a subtle perception. With practice you start identifying it. Fortunately, it is not necessary to perceive healing for the healing to work...after all, it's not about you! It's more about your pet's connection to Source, which you facilitate with your presence and gentle touch. It can help to inwardly notice *how* your pet is connected to Source. A purring cat or a relaxed dog can teach you a lot about this. Learn from them. Sense your own divinity, your own true nature, as a way to keep your heart open and your *Hara* quiet while your pet is receiving healing in their own way.

CHAPTER SEVEN

Common Mistakes & Myths

If you have read this far, you have the right motivation to learn this technique! There are hundreds of little tweaks that take place with your first few cancer cures. When I was first learning, every session had several "Ah-Ha!" moments as I "got it". I want that for you too, and I don't think I can teach it to you in a book. Some of it is so subtle that there needs to be an energetic attunement in order to learn it. Some of it is clarification of language. When we speak, one-on-one or with a group, we understand better.

Here are some common mistakes that we go through in the coaching:

- Magical Thinking versus careful observation of the four levels (physical, life force, emotional and spiritual).
- Pet too old.

- Confusing emotional flatness with objectivity and clear thinking. We discuss how to not lose our head when we turn on our heart and vice versa.

- Treating the cancer instead of the whole animal. You'll learn about Sam, a dog who should have been dead long ago, but is living healthy with "a touch of cancer".

- Pet with chemo/radiation. You'll learn how not to interfere with it if they are undergoing it, what to expect, what not to expect.

- Thinking you're a channel for Divine Love. You can think it—just don't confuse that with healing.

- Pet is on brink of death. You will meet Lady, a Border Collie who died from cancer 2 days after I met her. Tremendous meaning came from this. I have some ideas on how to save an animal in such a situation, but haven't had the resources to do it. Maybe together we will create what is needed for these situations.

- Too much regimentation. Cancer learns its way around just about anything. You have to keep changing. Lots of discussion on how to do this.

- Hating or loving the cancer. Detachment works better. You'll learn what to do with your hate or your love so it doesn't interfere with the healing.

- Avoiding the physical, nutritional, and Life Force levels. Sometimes the spiritual healing works by giving you the idea to change the diet, or something else. Sometimes money or time or resources open up — it's important to act on the inspiration you get.

- Fasting and/or dehydration inhibit this method of energy healing.

- Perfection paralysis. Take advantage of beginners luck and let me help you get started! Once you are cooling down the tumor, your confidence to proceed will grow. Don't wait for confidence to get started—that's putting the cart before the horse.

- Feeling that you have to be holy or enlightened or morally pure to cure cancer in your pet. It's best just to be yourself—warts and all.

- Insisting on treating an animal that doesn't like it. I can help you tweak your technique so you are not inadvertently "forcing" it upon your pet. If your pet doesn't want the healing, it won't work to insist.

CHAPTER EIGHT

Reasons *Why* People Stop

Good Reasons to Stop Treating

The best reason to stop treating your animal friend is if they are not "receiving" the treatments. There is no sense of "flow". They don't eat better, drink better, or sleep better. Their tumor doesn't cool down. The "nothing" you feel when you treat is really just that, with no sense that anything is happening at all. This could be an issue with your technique, so get support if you don't want to give up.

Another really good reason is if they are actively dying. There is an unconscious wisdom and order to the dying process. An animal's body *knows* how to die. It's best to go with the dying process rather than against it. It can be very beautiful. You can prolong their suffering if you are busy trying to get them to live. My method does not work if the animal is past their normal life span.

I can support you and them with my animal communication skills and distance healing to help them through their transition.

Sometimes, your pet may respond well to many treatments a day—more than you can comfortably give. A little sacrifice for your beloved companion is good, but you have to draw a line somewhere. Get help or let go if it is just too much for you. If this is you, before you give up, I hope we talk as I may be able to help you be just as effective without it taking so much time.

The "Other" Reasons

Then, there are also some reasons people use to stop – but have nothing to do with the treatment not working:

Lack of confidence. No one is confident their first or even second cancer cure! I can support you through this.

Lack of belief. This one surprises me as a reason people quit because belief is not required—none at all! If you believed that this would work, if you're really hunkered down and tried to get aligned with it, and it just isn't working, I would say, "Good!" Belief is not working. Now, you are ready to let go of belief and do the next step, which is more likely to work. *Simply carefully observe.* Keep belief and disbelief in a separate compartment from your work with your animal. You do need to keep your head in the game with interest. You do need to keep your curiosity alive so you can observe how your pet responds. That is not the same thing as psychically aligning with the method. You won't be able to tweak your technique if you believe you are doing it already. It's OK to believe in a possibility that you want to invite into your reality, but when that possibility starts getting close, its form shifts, and you can miss what is right under your nose if you are busy believing your original assumption. Keep it simple. Do not believe; just observe.

Peer pressure, especially from family. One of the reasons I like teaching pet owners is there is a lot less pressure from families to use chemo or radiation. It is often easier to simply follow your intuition and do what feels important and right to you, no matter what others think.

Philosophic pressure. This is pioneering work. It is not mainstream. The paradigm around cancer is shifting and there is a lot of resistance! You wouldn't be human if you didn't experience some of our culture's limitations inside you.

"It's taking too long." My hamster, Georgette was cured in about five 5-minutes sessions a week. It took about two weeks to go from lying still, almost dead in her cage, to full activity. It took another month for her hair to grow back where she lost it. She seemed fine so I didn't treat her much at all that month. See my YouTube video *Hamster Healed with Energy Medicine* that documented her cure. The dogs and cats I have worked with took much longer—months of daily 5-15 minute sessions by their owners. It's not really about size of animal, though that may be part of it. A larger animal could get better very quickly, or take months and months. If you pet is robustly responding to the sessions, I would encourage you to keep going. It doesn't hurt, it might save their life, and you spend some quality time with them.

Fear of Failure. Sometimes we don't give something our all because it is our last resource and we feel we can't cope if it doesn't work and we are faced with the fact that we have done everything we know. Get support.

Fear of Success. If this does work…if your pet does cure their cancer with your help…what does that mean for you? You will still be yourself. You will still have loads of human issues to work through. You will not be enlightened.   You will probably be super relieved and happy, and you might also experience a host of other emotions. When I had my first cure it rocked my inner world. As much as I wanted it, I felt that I had broken some "rule" that said it is impossible to cure cancer. I had to come to terms with the fact that what happened really happened. I had followed Bill Bengston's instructions, got some coaching, and the cancer went away. I had to work through its meaning in my life.   I'm still doing that. You will do it in your way. I am here if you need help.

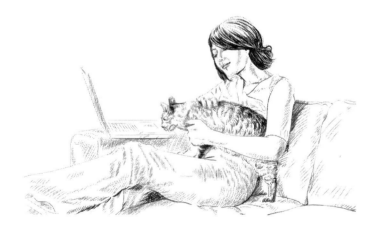

Relaxed video coaching

CHAPTER NINE

Your Next Step

At this point, you probably have lots of questions. Rather than describing my constantly evolving programs, I would like to invite you to have a conversation with me to decide how best to proceed. We can discuss what class, recording, book, energetically charted cotton, online group video class, one-to-one Skype session and distance healing options would suit your situation.

Simply email me at *info@spiritgate.com* saying that you read this book and want help with your pet. My office will send you a link to my online scheduler. There is no charge for this 10-15 minute "get acquainted" call. I want to make sure you are in the right place before you join one of my programs. You can also email and request website links that describe my current programs.

It would be my honor and pleasure to help you help your animal friend.

About the Author

Suzanne Clegg is a pioneer in holistic healthcare. Her 35-year career includes being a Licensed Acupuncturist, a Registered Dietitian Nutritionist, an herbalist and Medical Intuitive. She has four years graduate training in neurophysiology and is former Senior Faculty of the Acutonics® Institute of Integrative medicine. She was personally and extensively mentored by William Bengston, PhD in his healing method.

She has developed her own style of teaching pet owners to work with their pets with cancer. She combines distance healing with coaching pet owners to do a simple energy medicine technique to comfort and extend the life of their beloved animal friend.

She sees human patients in her private practice, Spirit Gate Acupuncture PC, in Lynbrook, New York where she also lives with her husband, daughter, and dog.

For more information, go to *www.SpiritGate.com*.

33128838R00038

Made in the USA
Middletown, DE
01 July 2016